DEALING WITH MALNUTRICTION
A TO Z
BY TAYLOR JONES

Introduction to Malnutrition

Malnutrition stands as a critical global health issue with far-reaching consequences that affect individuals, communities, and nations. Defined as a condition resulting from an imbalance between the body's nutrient needs and intake, malnutrition encompasses a spectrum of deficiencies and excesses in essential nutrients. This imbalance can lead to adverse physical, cognitive, and developmental outcomes, impacting the well-being of individuals across all age groups. In this exploration of malnutrition, we delve into its various forms, underlying causes, widespread effects, and the multifaceted efforts aimed at prevention and intervention. By understanding the complex interplay of factors contributing to malnutrition, we can better appreciate the urgency of addressing this challenge and developing sustainable solutions to ensure a healthier future for all.

Chapter 1

Definition of Malnutrition:

Malnutrition refers to a condition where there is an imbalance between the intake of nutrients and the body's nutritional requirements, leading to adverse health effects. It can manifest as deficiencies, excesses, or imbalances of essential nutrients such as proteins, carbohydrates, fats, vitamins, and minerals. Malnutrition encompasses both undernutrition, where the body does not receive sufficient nutrients, and overnutrition, where there is an excessive intake of certain nutrients, often accompanied by inadequate overall nutrition.

Importance of Adequate Nutrition

Adequate nutrition is a fundamental pillar of overall health and well-being. It plays a vital role in sustaining bodily functions, promoting growth and development, and safeguarding against a wide range of diseases and health complications. The significance of adequate nutrition becomes even more evident when considering the pervasive and far-reaching effects of malnutrition on individuals and societies.

1. **Physical Health**:

Adequate nutrition provides the body with the essential nutrients it needs to function optimally. Nutrients such as proteins, carbohydrates, fats, vitamins, and minerals are the building blocks of cells, tissues, and organs. They support processes like metabolism, immune response, and organ function. Insufficient intake of nutrients can weaken the immune system, making individuals more susceptible to infections and diseases. Conversely, a well-balanced diet strengthens the body's ability to fight off illnesses and recover from injuries.

2. **Growth and Development**:

Nutrition is particularly crucial during periods of rapid growth, such as childhood and adolescence. Proper nutrition ensures that children reach their full genetic potential in terms of height, weight, and cognitive development. Adequate intake of nutrients like protein, calcium, and vitamins supports bone growth, brain development, and cognitive function. Malnutrition during these critical phases can lead to stunted growth, developmental delays, and learning difficulties.

3. **Cognitive Function**:

Nutrition directly impacts cognitive function and brain health. Essential fatty acids, vitamins, and minerals are essential for maintaining proper brain structure and function. Omega-3 fatty acids, for example, are known to support cognitive processes and mood regulation. Malnutrition, particularly deficiencies in key nutrients like iron and iodine, can impair cognitive development, leading to decreased concentration, learning disabilities, and lower academic performance.

4. **Pregnancy and Maternal Health**:

Adequate nutrition is vital for pregnant women to support the health of both the mother and the developing fetus. Insufficient nutrition during pregnancy can result in preterm birth, low birth weight, and birth defects. Maternal malnutrition can also lead to long-term health risks for both the mother and child, such as an increased risk of chronic diseases later in life.

5. **Economic and Societal Impact**:

Malnutrition has significant economic implications for societies. Productivity losses due to malnutrition-related health issues can hinder economic growth. Moreover, the burden of treating malnutrition-related illnesses places strain on healthcare systems and resources.

Global Impact and Prevalence of Malnutrition

Malnutrition is a pressing global health issue that affects individuals, communities, and countries across the world. Its impact is multifaceted, ranging from individual health to economic development and social well-being. Understanding the prevalence and consequences of malnutrition on a global scale is crucial for implementing effective interventions and policies to address this challenge.

1. **Prevalence of Malnutrition**:

Malnutrition exists in various forms across all regions of the world. Both undernutrition and overnutrition are prevalent, contributing to a complex landscape of nutritional challenges.

Undernutrition: In low-income and middle-income countries, undernutrition remains a critical concern, particularly among children and pregnant women. According to the World Health Organization WHO, an estimated 144 million children under the age of five were stunted too short for their age in 2020.

Overnutrition: Overnutrition, characterized by obesity and diet-related non-communicable diseases, is on the rise globally. In 2020, more than 1.9 billion adults were overweight, with over 650 million being obese, according to the WHO.

2. **Health Consequences**:

The health consequences of malnutrition are far-reaching. Undernutrition can lead to weakened immune systems, making individuals more susceptible to infections and diseases. It can also result in stunted growth, cognitive impairments, and developmental delays in children. Overnutrition, on the other hand, increases the risk of chronic diseases such as diabetes, cardiovascular diseases, and certain types of cancer.

3. **Socioeconomic Impact**:

Malnutrition has profound socioeconomic implications. It hampers economic development by reducing productivity and increasing healthcare costs. In low-income and middle-income countries, the cycle of malnutrition and poverty often reinforces each other, as undernourished individuals are less likely to reach their full potential in terms of education and employment opportunities.

4. **Interconnected Factors**:

Malnutrition is driven by a complex interplay of factors. These include inadequate access to nutritious food, lack of education about proper nutrition, poverty, limited healthcare access, and cultural practices. Conflict, displacement, and climate change also contribute to malnutrition by disrupting food systems and livelihoods.

5. **Global Initiatives**:

International organizations and initiatives are working to combat malnutrition. The United Nations' Sustainable Development Goals SDGs include targets to end malnutrition in all its forms by 2030. Organizations like UNICEF, the World Food Program, and the World Health Organization collaborate with governments, NGOs, and communities to implement nutrition-focused interventions and programs.

6. **Future Challenges and Opportunities**:

Addressing malnutrition requires a comprehensive and integrated approach. This includes improving access to nutritious foods, promoting nutrition education, supporting breastfeeding, enhancing agricultural practices, and fostering multisectoral collaboration. Technological innovations, such as fortified foods and precision agriculture, hold promise in tackling malnutrition challenges.

Chapter2

Causes of Malnutrition

Malnutrition is caused by a complex interplay of factors that can vary across individuals, communities, and regions. The underlying causes of malnutrition are multifaceted and often interlinked, contributing to the wide range of nutritional deficiencies and imbalances observed worldwide.

1. **Insufficient Dietary Intake**:

Inadequate consumption of essential nutrients is a primary cause of malnutrition. This can occur due to several reasons:

Poverty: Limited financial resources can restrict access to a diverse and nutritious diet.

Food Insecurity: Inconsistent access to food due to factors like seasonal changes, natural disasters, or economic instability can lead to insufficient intake.

Limited Food Choices: Lack of availability and affordability of nutritious foods can result in reliance on cheaper, calorie-dense but nutrient-poor options.

2. **Poor Nutrient Absorption**:

Even when adequate nutrients are consumed, certain medical conditions can impair the body's ability to absorb and utilize them effectively:

Gastrointestinal Disorders: Conditions like celiac disease, Crohn's disease, and irritable bowel syndrome can hinder nutrient absorption.

Malabsorption Syndromes: Disorders that affect the absorption of specific nutrients, such as vitamin B12 or iron, can result in deficiencies.

3. **Medical Conditions and Diseases**:

Various health conditions can contribute to malnutrition:

Chronic Illness: Diseases like cancer, HIV/AIDS, and kidney disease increase the body's nutritional requirements and can lead to malnutrition.

Eating Disorders: Conditions such as anorexia nervosa and bulimia can result in severe nutrient deficiencies due to restricted food intake.

Infections: Illnesses that affect the gastrointestinal tract can disrupt nutrient absorption and lead to malnutrition.

4. **Lack of Access to Clean Water and Sanitation**:

Unsafe drinking water and poor sanitation contribute to infections and diseases that can impair nutrient absorption and increase nutrient requirements.

5. **Dietary Practices and Cultural Factors**:

Cultural beliefs, taboos, and traditional dietary practices can impact nutritional intake:

Early Introduction of Complementary Foods: Inappropriate introduction of solid foods to infants can lead to deficiencies in vital nutrients.

Food Taboos: Certain cultural restrictions on certain foods can limit nutrient intake.

6. **Gender Inequality**:

In many societies, women and girls may have restricted access to food and nutrition due to unequal distribution within households.

7. **Lack of Nutrition Education**:

Lack of knowledge about balanced diets, optimal feeding practices, and the importance of diverse foods can contribute to malnutrition.

8. **Socioeconomic Factors**:

Social and economic disparities play a significant role in malnutrition:

Income Inequality: Poorer communities may have limited access to nutritious foods and healthcare.

Lack of Education: Limited education can hinder understanding of proper nutrition and health practices.

9. **Environmental Factors**:

Environmental conditions such as climate change, natural disasters, and loss of biodiversity can impact food production, availability, and nutrient content.

10. **Globalization and Urbanization**:

Rapid urbanization and changing lifestyles can lead to shifts in dietary patterns, often favoring calorie-dense, nutrient-poor foods.

Addressing malnutrition requires a comprehensive approach that takes into account the diverse factors contributing to its occurrence. This includes improving access to nutritious foods, promoting education about healthy eating habits, enhancing healthcare services, and addressing underlying social and economic inequalities.

Chapter 3

Types of Malnutrition:

Undernutrition and Overnutrition

1. **Undernutrition /Undernourishment**:

Undernutrition refers to a state where an individual's dietary intake fails to meet their body's energy and nutrient requirements. It is characterized by deficiencies in essential nutrients such as calories, proteins, vitamins, and minerals. Undernutrition can take several forms:

Protein-Energy Malnutrition PEM: This is one of the most severe forms of undernutrition. It occurs when there is a deficiency of both calories and protein. PEM includes two distinct conditions: marasmus and kwashiorkor.

Marasmus: Marasmus is characterized by severe wasting of muscle and body fat, resulting in a thin and emaciated appearance. Children with marasmus often have very low weight for their age and may experience growth retardation.

Kwashiorkor: Kwashiorkor is characterized by protein deficiency, often seen in children who have access to some calories but lack sufficient protein intake. Symptoms may include swelling (edema) in the abdomen and limbs, fatty liver, and changes in hair and skin pigmentation.

Stunting: Stunting occurs when a child's height is significantly below the average for their age due to chronic undernutrition. Stunting is an indicator of long-term nutritional deficiencies and is associated with impaired physical and cognitive development.

Wasting: Wasting is characterized by a low weight for height, often due to acute food shortage or illness. It signifies recent weight loss and is an indicator of acute undernutrition.

Micronutrient Deficiencies: Undernutrition can lead to deficiencies in essential vitamins and minerals such as iron, vitamin A, iodine, and zinc. These deficiencies can result in a range of health issues, including anemia, impaired vision, compromised immune function, and developmental delays.

2. **Overnutrition/Overeating**:

Overnutrition, also known as overeating, occurs when individuals consistently consume more calories than their bodies need for energy expenditure and growth. This excess caloric intake can lead to overweight and obesity. Overnutrition is commonly associated with diets high in calorie-dense, nutrient-poor foods, often rich in sugars, unhealthy fats, and refined carbohydrates. Key aspects of overnutrition include:

Obesity: Obesity is a condition where an individual's body mass index BMI is significantly above the healthy range. It is a major risk factor for various chronic diseases, including type 2 diabetes, cardiovascular diseases, and certain cancers.

Metabolic Syndrome: Overnutrition contributes to the development of metabolic syndrome, a cluster of conditions including high blood pressure, elevated blood sugar levels, high cholesterol, and excess abdominal fat. These factors increase the risk of heart disease and diabetes.

Non-Communicable Diseases NCDs: Overnutrition is a major contributor to the rise of non-communicable diseases, which are long-term health conditions that are often preventable and influenced by lifestyle factors. NCDs include heart disease, stroke, diabetes, and certain types of cancer.

Addressing both undernutrition and overnutrition requires a multi-pronged approach that focuses on education, access to nutritious foods, public health interventions, and policy changes. A balanced and varied diet, along with healthy lifestyle choices, is essential to ensure proper nutritional status and prevent the adverse health effects associated with both types of malnutrition.

Chapter 4

Effects of Malnutrition

Malnutrition, whether due to undernutrition or overnutrition, has far-reaching and often devastating effects on the health and well-being of individuals. These effects can impact various aspects of physical, cognitive, and overall development, with implications for individuals and societies as a whole.

1. **Physical Health Consequences**:

Undernutrition:

Stunted Growth: Insufficient intake of calories and nutrients during critical growth phases, such as childhood and adolescence, can lead to stunted growth, where individuals fail to reach their full genetic height potential.

Weak Immune System: Undernourished individuals have weakened immune systems, making them more susceptible to infections, illnesses, and slower recovery.

Muscle Wasting: Protein-energy malnutrition can result in muscle wasting, leading to reduced strength and physical capabilities.

Anemia: Iron deficiency can lead to anemia, characterized by fatigue, weakness, and decreased oxygen-carrying capacity of the blood.

Bone Health Issues: Inadequate calcium and vitamin D intake can impair bone health, increasing the risk of fractures and osteoporosis.

⊥ Overnutrition:

Obesity: Excessive calorie intake leads to obesity, which increases the risk of chronic diseases like type 2 diabetes, heart disease, stroke, and certain types of cancer.

Cardiovascular Issues: Overnutrition contributes to high blood pressure, elevated cholesterol levels, and atherosclerosis, which can result in heart attacks and strokes.

Type 2 Diabetes: Overeating, especially foods high in refined sugars and unhealthy fats, can lead to insulin resistance and the development of type 2 diabetes.

Joint Problems: Excess weight puts strain on joints, leading to conditions such as osteoarthritis.

Liver and Kidney Diseases: Overnutrition, especially in the form of high-sugar diets, can contribute to fatty liver disease and kidney problems.

2. **Cognitive and Developmental Effects**:

⊥ Undernutrition:

Cognitive Impairment: Malnourished children often experience cognitive deficits, including reduced attention span, memory problems, and lower IQ scores.

Learning Disabilities: Chronic undernutrition can lead to learning disabilities and developmental delays, affecting academic performance and overall cognitive development.

- **Overnutrition**:

Cognitive Decline: Obesity and overnutrition are linked to cognitive decline and an increased risk of neurodegenerative diseases like Alzheimer's disease.

Mental Health: Overnutrition can impact mental health, contributing to conditions like depression and anxiety.

3. **Impact on Immune System**:

Undernutrition: Undernutrition weakens the immune system's ability to fight infections, making individuals more susceptible to diseases and prolonging recovery times.

Overnutrition: Overnutrition can lead to chronic inflammation, which negatively affects immune function and increases the risk of infections and autoimmune disorders.

4. **Reproductive and Maternal Health**:

Undernutrition: Malnutrition during pregnancy can result in low birth weight, preterm birth, and developmental issues in the child. It also increases the risk of maternal complications during childbirth.

Overnutrition: Obesity can lead to complications during pregnancy, including gestational diabetes and hypertension. It also increases the risk of birth defects and future health issues for both the mother and child.

5. **Long-Term Health Risks**:

Both undernutrition and overnutrition during critical developmental periods can have lasting effects on health into adulthood, increasing the risk of chronic diseases and reducing overall life expectancy.

Chapter 5

Malnutrition in Different Age Groups

Malnutrition affects individuals across all age groups, from infancy to old age. The specific nutritional needs and vulnerabilities of each age group contribute to distinct patterns of malnutrition and associated health risks.

1. **Infant and Child Malnutrition**:

Infants and young children are particularly susceptible to malnutrition due to their rapid growth and development. Key aspects include:

Undernutrition: Insufficient breastfeeding and inadequate introduction of appropriate complementary foods can lead to malnutrition. This may result in stunted growth, underweight, and micronutrient deficiencies.

Exclusive Breastfeeding: Lack of exclusive breastfeeding during the first six months of life can contribute to malnutrition. Breast milk provides essential nutrients and protects against infections.

Micronutrient Deficiencies: Young children are at risk of micronutrient deficiencies, particularly iron and vitamin A deficiencies, which can impair physical growth, immune function, and cognitive development.

2. **Adolescent Nutritional Challenges**:

Adolescents experience rapid growth, increased energy requirements, and changing dietary preferences. However, malnutrition can still affect this age group:

Unbalanced Diets: Adolescents may develop poor eating habits, opting for energy-dense but nutrient-poor foods high in sugars and unhealthy fats.

Micronutrient Needs: Adolescents require increased intake of nutrients like calcium for bone growth and development, iron for menstrual health, and vitamin D for bone health.

3. **Malnutrition in the Elderly**:

Older adults often face unique challenges related to nutrition and health:

Reduced Appetite: Loss of appetite and changes in metabolism can lead to inadequate nutrient intake among the elderly, increasing the risk of malnutrition.

Nutrient Absorption: Age-related changes in the digestive system can impair nutrient absorption, leading to deficiencies.

Frailty and Sarcopenia: Muscle loss (sarcopenia) and frailty are common issues in the elderly, often exacerbated by malnutrition and leading to functional decline.

Micronutrient Deficiencies: Older adults may face deficiencies in vitamins such as B12 and D, as well as minerals like calcium, which can impact bone health and overall well-being.

4. **Pregnancy and Lactation**:

Pregnant women and breastfeeding mothers have increased nutritional needs to support their own health and the growth of the fetus or infant:

Undernutrition: Inadequate nutrition during pregnancy can lead to low birth weight, preterm birth, and developmental issues in the child. Maternal malnutrition also increases the risk of complications during childbirth.

Micronutrient Needs: Adequate intake of folic acid, iron, calcium, and other vitamins and minerals is essential for maternal and fetal health.

5. **Athletes and Active Individuals**:

Individuals engaged in sports and physical activities have specific nutritional requirements:

Energy Balance: Athletes must balance energy expenditure with caloric intake to prevent undernutrition, which can impact performance and recovery.

Macronutrient Needs: Athletes require sufficient carbohydrates for energy, proteins for muscle repair and growth, and healthy fats for overall health.

Hydration: Adequate fluid intake is crucial to prevent dehydration, particularly during intense physical activity.

Understanding the unique nutritional needs of each age group and addressing these needs through appropriate dietary choices, supplementation, and healthcare interventions is essential for preventing malnutrition and promoting overall health and well-being.

Chapter 6

Malnutrition in Developing vs. Developed Countries

Malnutrition manifests differently in developing and developed countries due to varying socioeconomic factors, healthcare infrastructure, and access to resources. These disparities contribute to distinct patterns of malnutrition and associated challenges.

+ Malnutrition in Developing Countries:

1. **Undernutrition**: Developing countries often face higher prevalence of undernutrition due to poverty, limited access to food, and inadequate healthcare systems.

Stunting and Wasting: Chronic malnutrition, characterized by stunted growth and wasting, is more prevalent in developing countries, particularly among children. Limited access to nutrient-rich foods contributes to these issues.

Micronutrient Deficiencies: Deficiencies in essential vitamins and minerals, such as vitamin A, iron, and iodine, are common in developing countries. Lack of access to diverse diets and fortified foods contributes to these deficiencies.

2. **Food Insecurity**: Many developing countries struggle with food insecurity, where consistent access to nutritious and safe food is limited. This can result from poverty, political instability, conflicts, and climate-related challenges.

3. **Lack of Access to Clean Water and Sanitation**: Poor access to clean water and sanitation increases the risk of infections and diseases that worsen malnutrition.

4. **Limited Healthcare Infrastructure**: Developing countries often have inadequate healthcare systems, which hinders timely diagnosis and treatment of malnutrition-related health issues.

┿Malnutrition in Developed Countries:

1. **Overnutrition and Obesity**: Developed countries face a growing problem of overnutrition, particularly obesity, due to the availability of energy-dense, processed foods and sedentary lifestyles.

Unhealthy Diets: Diets high in unhealthy fats, sugars, and refined carbohydrates contribute to obesity and related health issues like type 2 diabetes and cardiovascular diseases.

Food Deserts and Poor Dietary Choices: Even in developed countries, there are areas with limited access to fresh, nutritious foods, known as "food deserts." This can lead to reliance on cheaper, processed foods.

2. **Nutrient Imbalances**: While overnutrition is a concern, certain nutrient imbalances can also affect developed countries:

Micronutrient Deficiencies: Even in countries with abundance of food, some individuals may have limited intake of nutrient-rich foods, leading to deficiencies in vitamins and minerals.

Excessive Consumption of Certain Nutrients: Paradoxically, certain populations in developed countries may consume excessive amounts of certain nutrients, leading to health risks.

For instance, excess sodium intake can contribute to hypertension.

3. **Sedentary Lifestyles**: Modern lifestyles in developed countries often involve sedentary behaviors, contributing to weight gain and obesity.

4. **Aging Populations**: Developed countries with aging populations face unique challenges, including malnutrition among the elderly due to reduced appetite, impaired nutrient absorption, and limited access to proper nutrition.

In both developing and developed countries, addressing malnutrition requires tailored approaches. In developing countries, efforts may focus on improving access to nutritious foods, promoting breastfeeding, implementing nutrition education programs, and enhancing healthcare systems. In developed countries, interventions may include promoting healthy eating habits, encouraging physical activity, regulating food advertising, and raising awareness about the risks of overnutrition. Recognizing the distinct challenges faced by each context is essential for effective strategies to combat malnutrition.

Chapter 7

Addressing and Preventing Malnutrition

Addressing and preventing malnutrition is a multifaceted endeavor that requires a combination of strategies, policies, and interventions at individual, community, and societal levels. These approaches vary based on the type of malnutrition, underlying causes, and the specific context. Here are some key ways to address and prevent malnutrition:

1. **Nutritional Education and Awareness**:

Public Health Campaigns: Government and non-governmental organizations can run campaigns to raise awareness about the importance of balanced diets, proper feeding practices, and the risks of both undernutrition and overnutrition.

School-based Programs: Incorporating nutrition education into school curricula helps children and adolescents learn about healthy eating habits from an early age.

2. **Access to Nutritious Food**:

Promote Breastfeeding: Encourage exclusive breastfeeding during the first six months of life and continued breastfeeding alongside complementary foods.

Community Gardens and Urban Farming: Support initiatives that promote local food production, which can increase access to fresh produce, especially in urban areas.

Food Subsidies: Governments can provide subsidies for nutrient-rich foods to make them more affordable for low-income populations.

Food Assistance Programs: Implement food assistance programs that provide nutritious foods to vulnerable populations, such as pregnant women, infants, and the elderly.

3. **Food Security and Sustainable Agriculture**:

Diversification of Crops: Encourage the cultivation of a diverse range of crops to ensure a varied and balanced diet.

Promote Agroecological Practices: Support sustainable and environmentally friendly farming practices that enhance soil fertility and preserve biodiversity.

4. **Healthcare Interventions**:

Nutritional Supplementation: Provide nutrient supplements, such as vitamin A capsules and iron tablets, to address specific deficiencies, especially in at-risk populations like children and pregnant women.

Treatment of Underlying Conditions: Address medical conditions that can lead to malnutrition, such as infections and digestive disorders.

5. **Government Policies and Regulation**:

Food Labeling: Enforce clear and informative food labeling to help consumers make informed choices about their food purchases.

Taxation and Regulation: Implement taxes on unhealthy foods and beverages high in sugars and unhealthy fats to discourage their consumption. Regulate advertising of such products, especially targeting children.

School Nutrition Programs: Establish and enforce guidelines for healthy foods in schools, ensuring that children have access to nutritious meals during school hours.

6. Research and Innovation:

Fortification of Foods: Fortify staple foods with essential vitamins and minerals to address micronutrient deficiencies.

Biofortification: Develop crops with enhanced nutritional content to address specific nutrient deficiencies in regions with limited dietary diversity.

Nutrition Monitoring: Establish robust systems for monitoring the nutritional status of populations to identify trends and target interventions effectively.

7. Behavioral Change:

Counseling and Support: Provide counseling and support to individuals and families, helping them adopt healthy eating habits and lifestyles.

Promotion of Physical Activity: Encourage regular physical activity as a complement to healthy eating to prevent overnutrition and obesity.

Addressing and preventing malnutrition requires a comprehensive approach that takes into account the diverse factors contributing to its occurrence. It involves collaboration among governments, international organizations, healthcare professionals, educators, communities, and individuals. By combining efforts across multiple fronts, societies can work towards reducing the prevalence of malnutrition and improving overall health outcomes.

Chapter 8

Case Studies and Global Initiatives

1. Scaling Up Nutrition SUN Movement:

The Scaling Up Nutrition SUN Movement is a global initiative launched in 2010 to combat malnutrition in all its forms. It brings together governments, civil society, the United Nations, donors, businesses, and researchers to coordinate efforts and share best practices. SUN focuses on supporting countries in developing and implementing multi-sectoral nutrition plans that address the underlying causes of malnutrition.

TAYLOR JONES

2. **Community-Based Management of Acute Malnutrition CMAM:**

CMAM is a widely recognized approach for treating severe acute malnutrition SAM in resource-limited settings. It involves identifying and treating children with SAM through community health workers, therapeutic feeding centers, and outpatient programs. By providing ready-to-use therapeutic foods and closely monitoring progress, CMAM has been effective in reducing mortality rates among malnourished children.

3. **Golden Rice:**

Golden Rice is a genetically modified rice variety developed to address vitamin A deficiency, particularly in developing countries where rice is a staple food. It is engineered to produce beta-carotene, a precursor to vitamin A. By consuming Golden Rice, populations that rely heavily on rice can potentially improve their vitamin A intake and reduce related health risks.

4. **Alive & Thrive:**

TAYLOR JONES

Alive & thrive is an initiative focused on improving infant and young child feeding practices to prevent undernutrition. It has implemented programs in several countries, promoting exclusive breastfeeding, timely introduction of complementary foods, and proper nutrition during the first 1,000 days of life.

5. **World Food Program WFP**:

The WFP, a United Nations agency, provides food assistance to vulnerable populations, especially during emergencies. It also implements long-term initiatives to improve access to nutritious foods, such as school feeding programs that not only alleviate hunger but also encourage school attendance and retention.

6. **National Nutrition Mission POSHAN Abhiyaan - India**:

India's National Nutrition Mission, also known as POSHAN Abhiyaan, aims to improve nutritional outcomes for children, pregnant women, and lactating mothers. It focuses on preventing and reducing undernutrition and low birth weight through a multi-sectoral approach that includes nutrition interventions, health services, sanitation, and hygiene.

7. **Nutrition-Sensitive Agriculture Programs**:

Several initiatives focus on integrating nutrition into agricultural practices. For example, the Biofortification Challenge seeks to develop crops with enhanced nutrient content, addressing micronutrient deficiencies directly through food sources.

8. Scaling Up Nutrition Business Network SBN:

The SBN brings together businesses from different sectors to collaborate on improving nutrition. It encourages companies to adopt practices that promote healthy food production, marketing, and distribution, contributing to better food choices and nutritional outcomes.

9. EAT-Lancet Commission:

The EAT-Lancet Commission is a global initiative that addresses both health and environmental sustainability. It offers dietary guidelines that aim to provide nutritious and sustainable diets for the world's growing population while minimizing the environmental impact of food production.

These case studies and initiatives showcase the diverse approaches taken to address malnutrition on a global scale. They emphasize the importance of multi-sectoral collaboration, innovation, education, and policy changes to achieve lasting improvements in nutritional status and overall health outcomes.

Chapter 9

Future Outlook and Trends in Malnutrition

As we look to the future, several key trends and developments are shaping the landscape of malnutrition prevention and management. These trends are influenced by factors such as technological advancements, changing dietary patterns, global health priorities, and environmental concerns. Understanding these trends is crucial for developing effective strategies to address malnutrition in the years to come.

1. **Double Burden of Malnutrition**:

The double burden of malnutrition refers to the coexistence of undernutrition and overnutrition within the same population or even the same individual. Many countries are grappling with the challenge of combating stunting and micronutrient deficiencies while simultaneously addressing rising rates of obesity and diet-related chronic diseases. Addressing this dual challenge requires nuanced interventions that consider both sides of the spectrum.

2. **Urbanization and Dietary Transitions**:

As populations increasingly move to urban areas, dietary patterns tend to shift towards more processed, calorie-dense, and nutrient-poor foods. Urbanization is associated with sedentary lifestyles and increased consumption of fast food and sugary beverages, contributing to rising rates of overweight, obesity, and diet-related diseases.

3. **Impact of Climate Change**:

Climate change poses a significant threat to food security and nutrition. Changes in temperature and precipitation patterns can disrupt agricultural production, affecting crop yields and food availability. This can lead to increased food prices and decreased access to nutritious foods, particularly in vulnerable communities.

4. **Nutritional Innovations**:

Advancements in biotechnology and food science are leading to innovations in nutrition. Biofortified crops, genetically modified organisms GMOs designed for enhanced nutrient content, and lab-grown meat are examples of innovations that could address nutritional deficiencies and sustainability challenges.

5. **Digital Health Solutions**:

Technology is playing a crucial role in providing health information and promoting behavior change. Mobile apps, wearable devices, and online platforms can help individuals track their nutritional intake, receive personalized dietary recommendations, and access nutrition education.

6. **Global Health Agendas**:

International initiatives and agendas, such as the United Nations' Sustainable Development Goals SDGs, continue to emphasize the importance of addressing malnutrition. These agendas set targets for improving nutrition, reducing stunting, and ending hunger by 2030.

7. **School Nutrition and Early Childhood Interventions**:

Investing in school nutrition programs and early childhood interventions can have lasting effects on reducing malnutrition. Nutritional interventions during critical developmental periods can support healthy growth and cognitive development, breaking the cycle of malnutrition.

8. **Policy Shifts and Regulatory Measures**:

Governments and health organizations are increasingly implementing policies to promote healthier diets. Sugar taxes, front-of-pack labeling, and restrictions on marketing unhealthy foods to children are some examples of regulatory measures aimed at combating overnutrition.

9. **Focus on Sustainability**:

The environmental impact of food production is becoming a critical consideration. Sustainable agriculture practices, reduction of food waste, and promoting plant-based diets are trends aligned with both nutrition and environmental goals.

10. **Resilience and Adaptation**:

Building resilience in communities vulnerable to malnutrition involves addressing social, economic, and environmental factors. This includes improving access to clean water, sanitation, education, and healthcare to mitigate the effects of malnutrition.

Conclusion

In conclusion, malnutrition remains a multifaceted global challenge that affects individuals, communities, and nations across the world. Whether characterized by undernutrition, overnutrition, or the dual burden of both, malnutrition has far-reaching implications for physical health, cognitive development, and overall well-being. The complex interplay of factors contributing to malnutrition—ranging from economic disparities and inadequate access to nutritious foods to changing dietary patterns and environmental concerns—underscores the need for comprehensive and tailored approaches to prevention and intervention.

The future outlook on malnutrition is marked by promising trends in nutrition education, technological innovations, sustainable agriculture, and the increasing alignment of global health agendas. These trends provide opportunities to address malnutrition holistically, emphasizing the importance of collaboration, policy reform, and behavior change. However, challenges such as climate change, urbanization, and the persistence of food insecurity necessitate ongoing vigilance and adaptability in our strategies.

As we move forward, it is crucial to recognize that addressing malnutrition requires a united effort from governments, organizations, healthcare professionals, educators, communities, and individuals. By embracing a multidimensional approach that integrates nutrition education, access to nutritious foods, healthcare interventions, and policy changes, societies can work toward a future where malnutrition is minimized, health disparities are reduced, and all individuals have the opportunity to lead healthier and more fulfilling lives. Through collective action, we can shape a future in which malnutrition is overcome, enabling communities to thrive and reach their full potential.